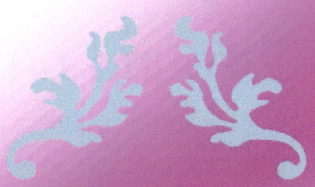

CANCER HAS MOMMA

A Life Skill Social Story about a Parent having Cancer

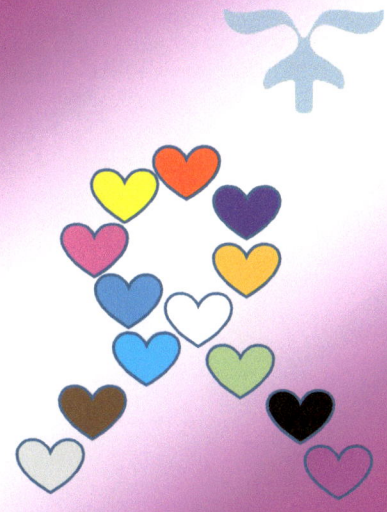

AUTHOR & ILLUSTRATED BY:
LAURA L. VERCILLO
A PACED PATIENCE BOOK

Momma has cancer. I was a little afraid when I found out.

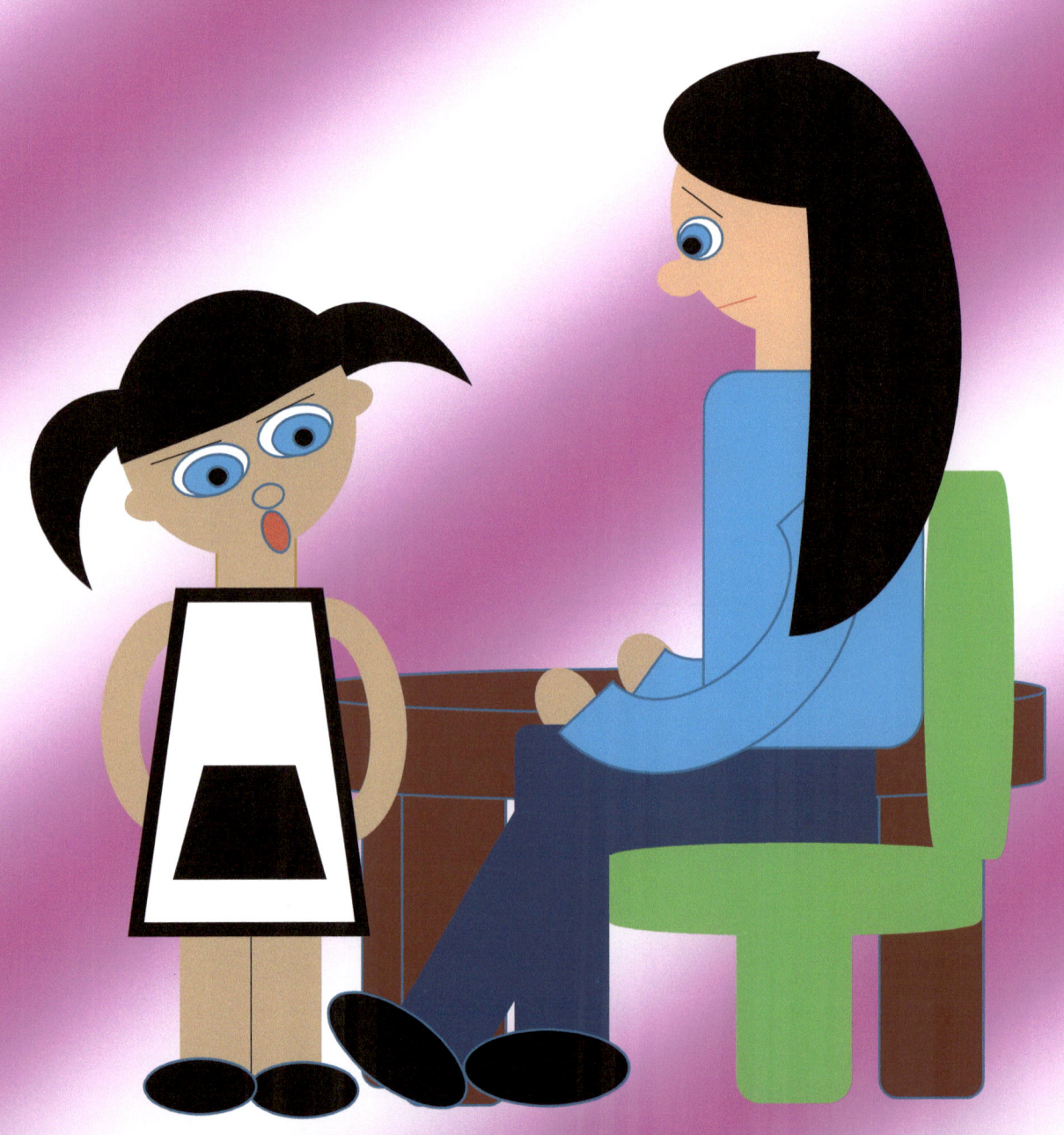

Ok, I was a lot afraid when I found out.

I thought Momma was going to die. I thought maybe I would get cancer too.

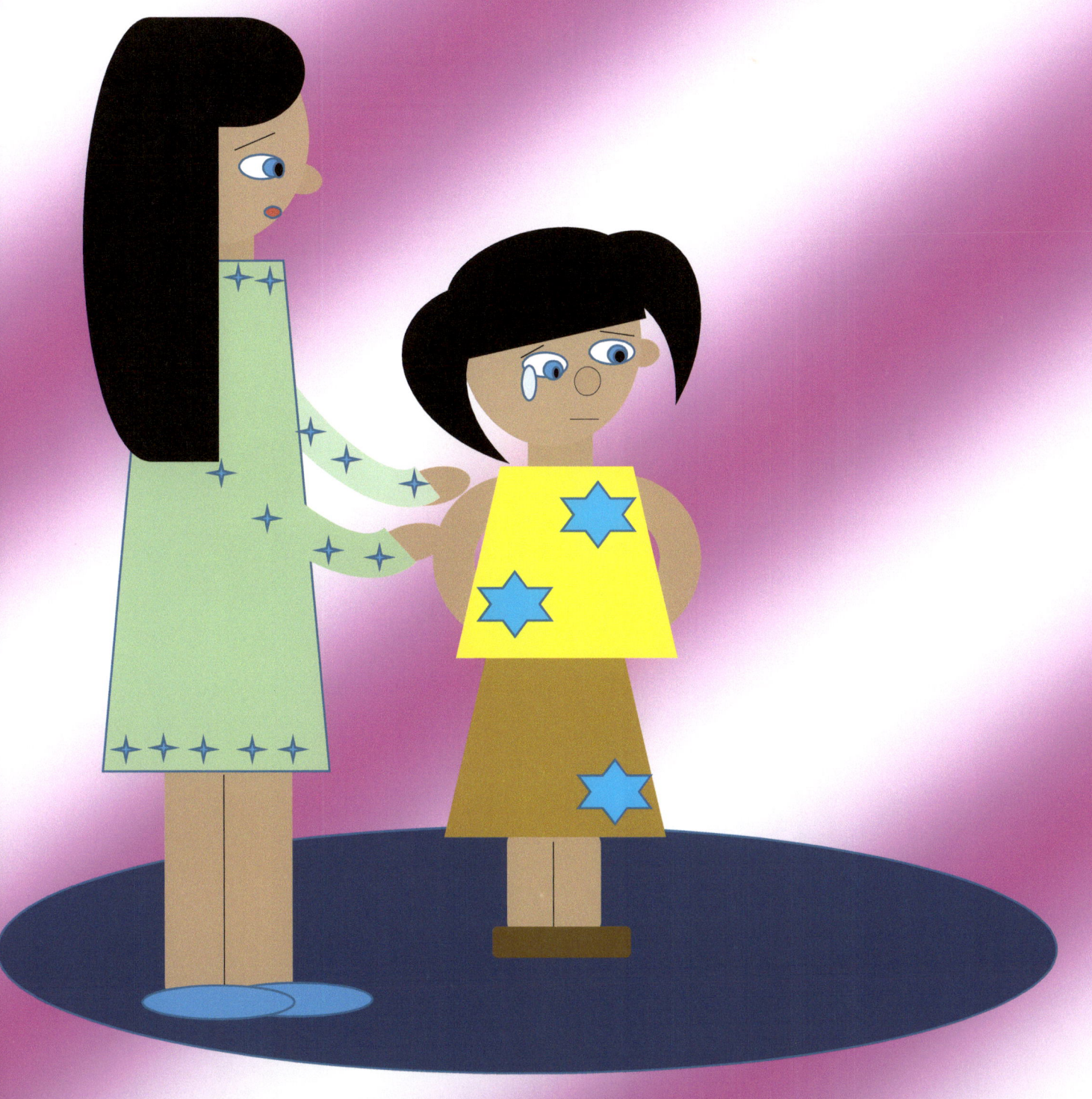

Cancer can grow in and on your body. Some people get cancer. Some people don't. It's not like a cold. You can't catch it.

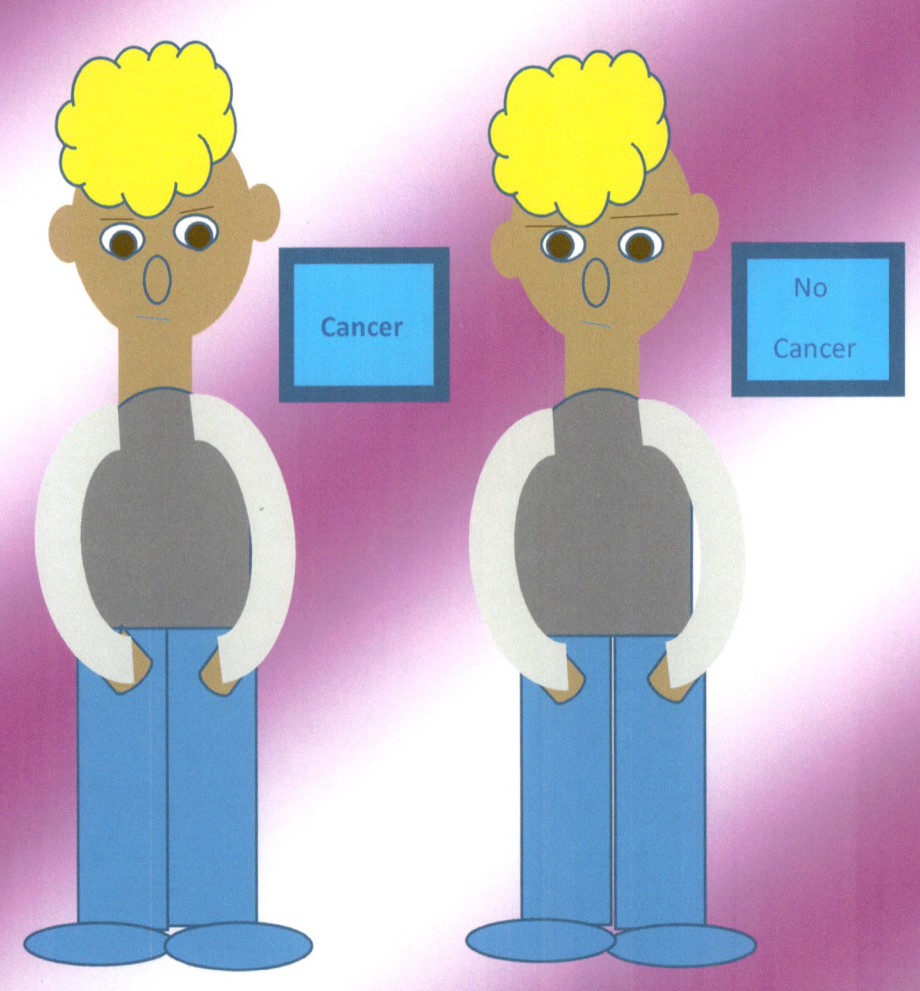

Momma had to go through a lot of tests. I learned about cancer. There are all kinds of types of cancers. They have long names and I can't say them all. Cancer is different for everyone.

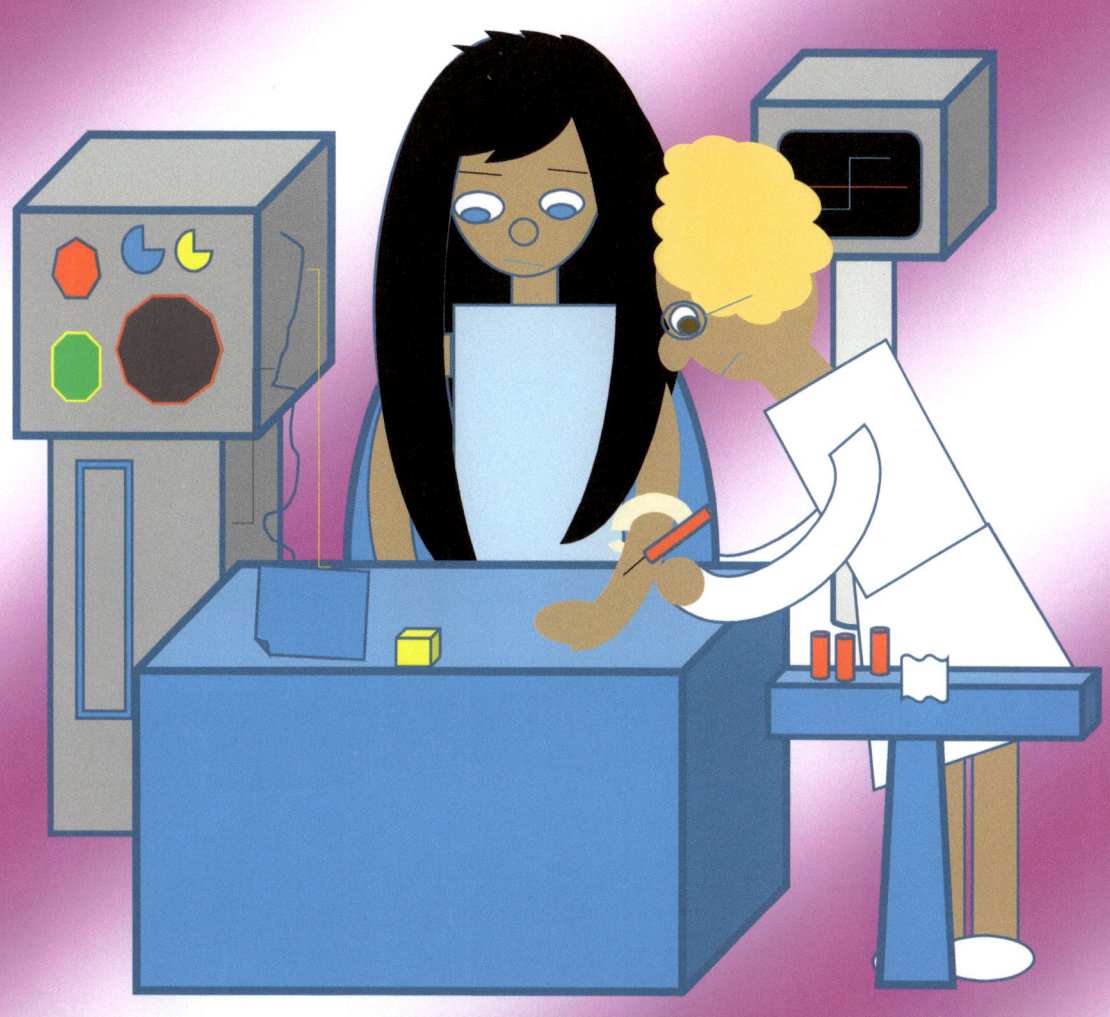

Cancer is not easy. It can make you real sick. Sometimes the medicine she takes for the cancer makes her sick too.

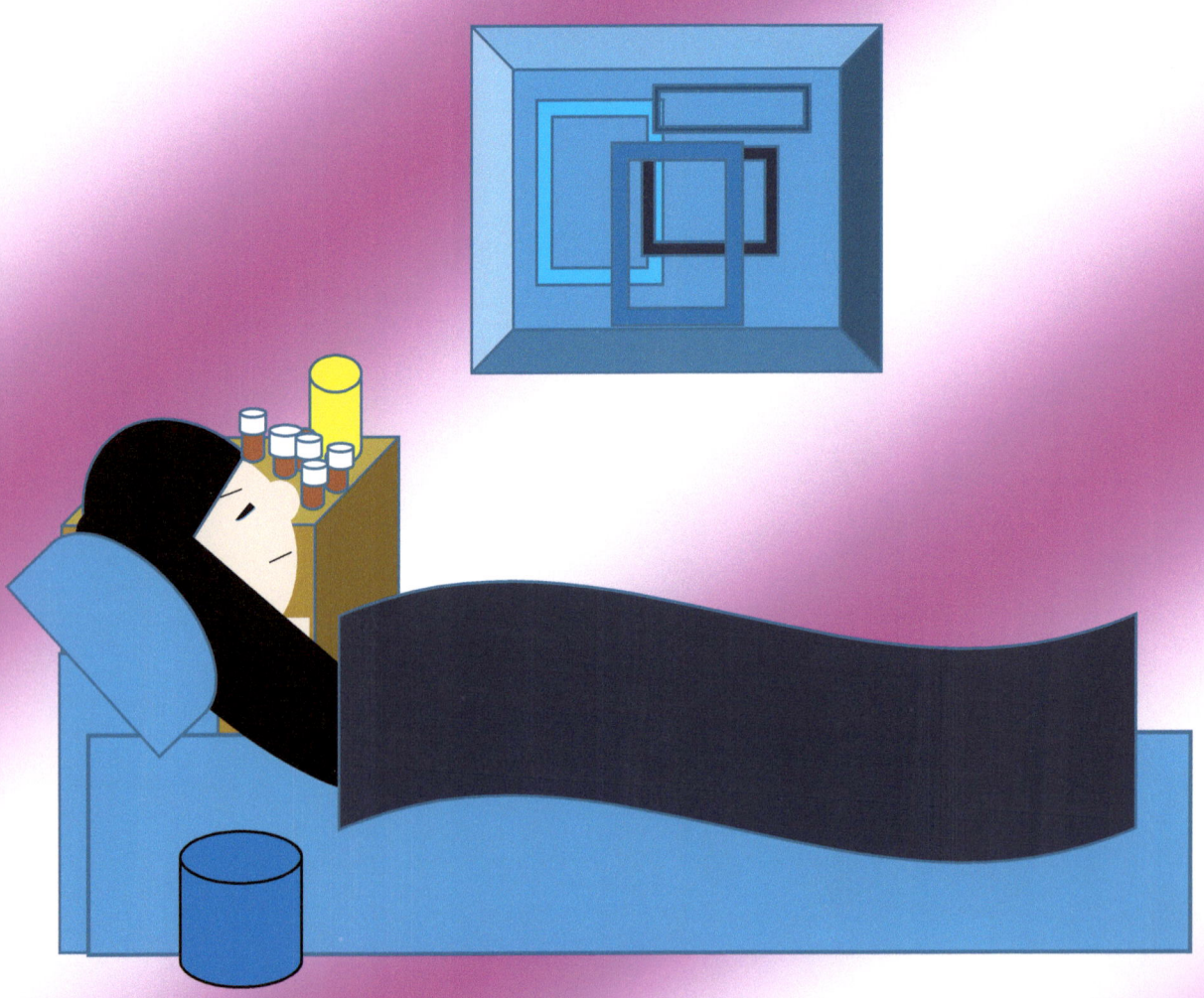

Cancer takes away things from momma. Sometimes it's her time, her happy face, or her energy. It stole all her hair.

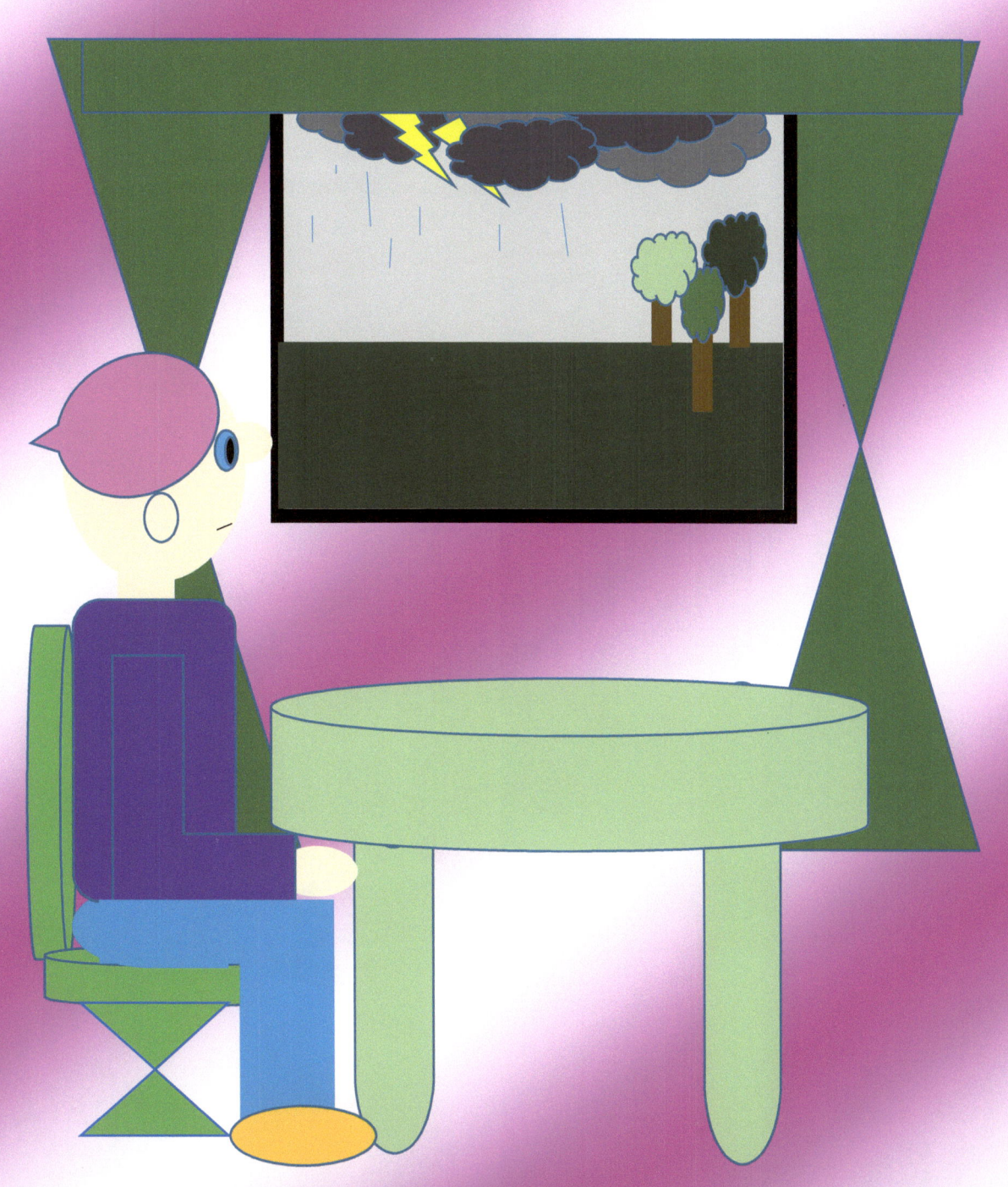

One thing cancer can't take is her love for us.

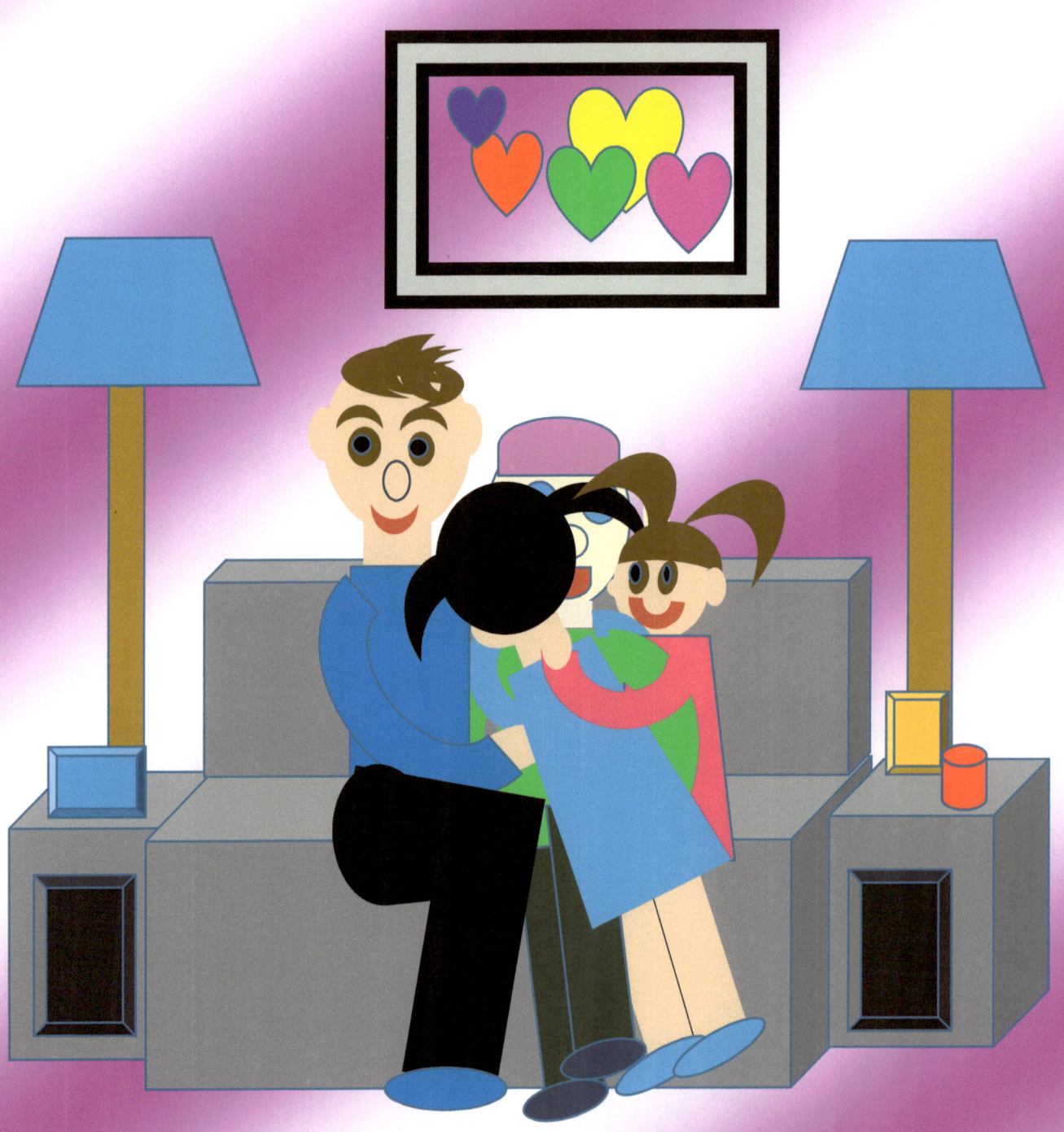

I cried and so did Momma. I just felt sad. Momma is beautiful with or without hair. I now know she is beautiful inside. Outside is nice, but it's her inside that makes her so beautiful!

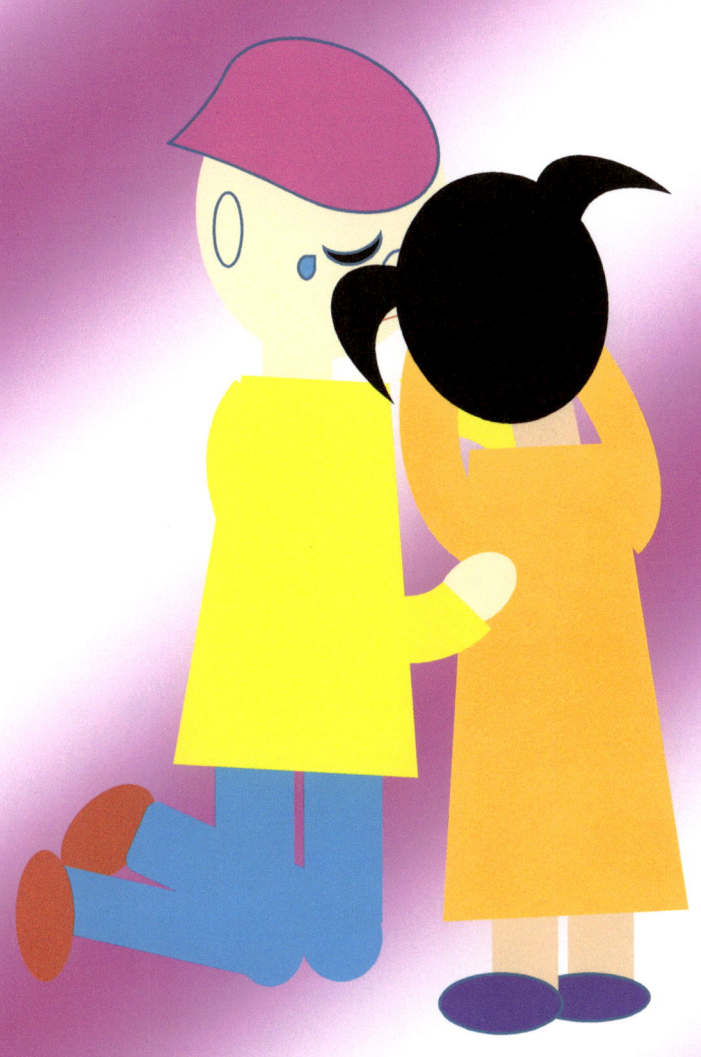

Momma says I am a big help. Sometimes I help by watching my little sister. Sometimes I help by just holding momma's hand.

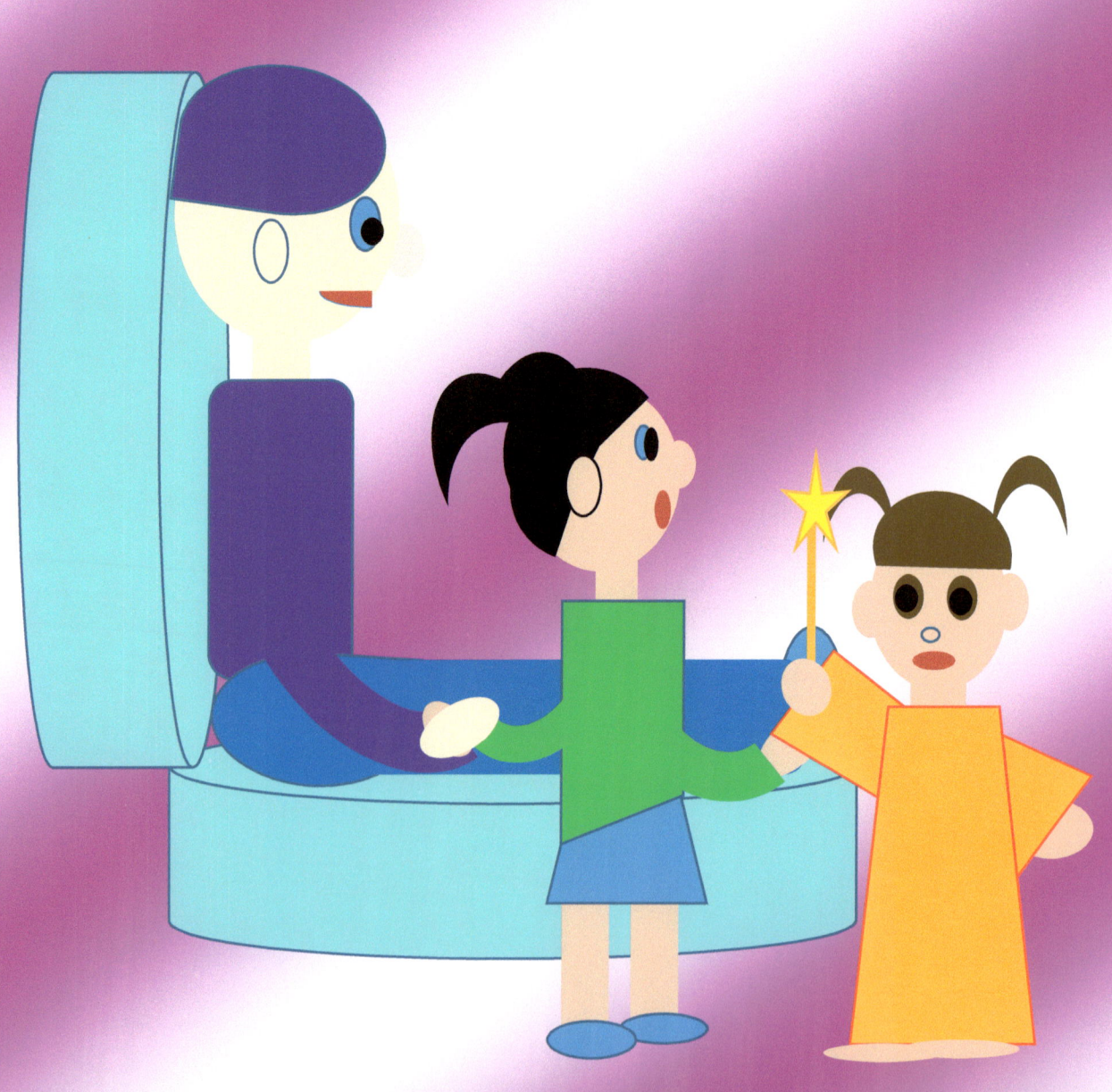

We need to make sure the house stays clean for momma. Her immunity is low during her treatment. She can get sick easier right now.

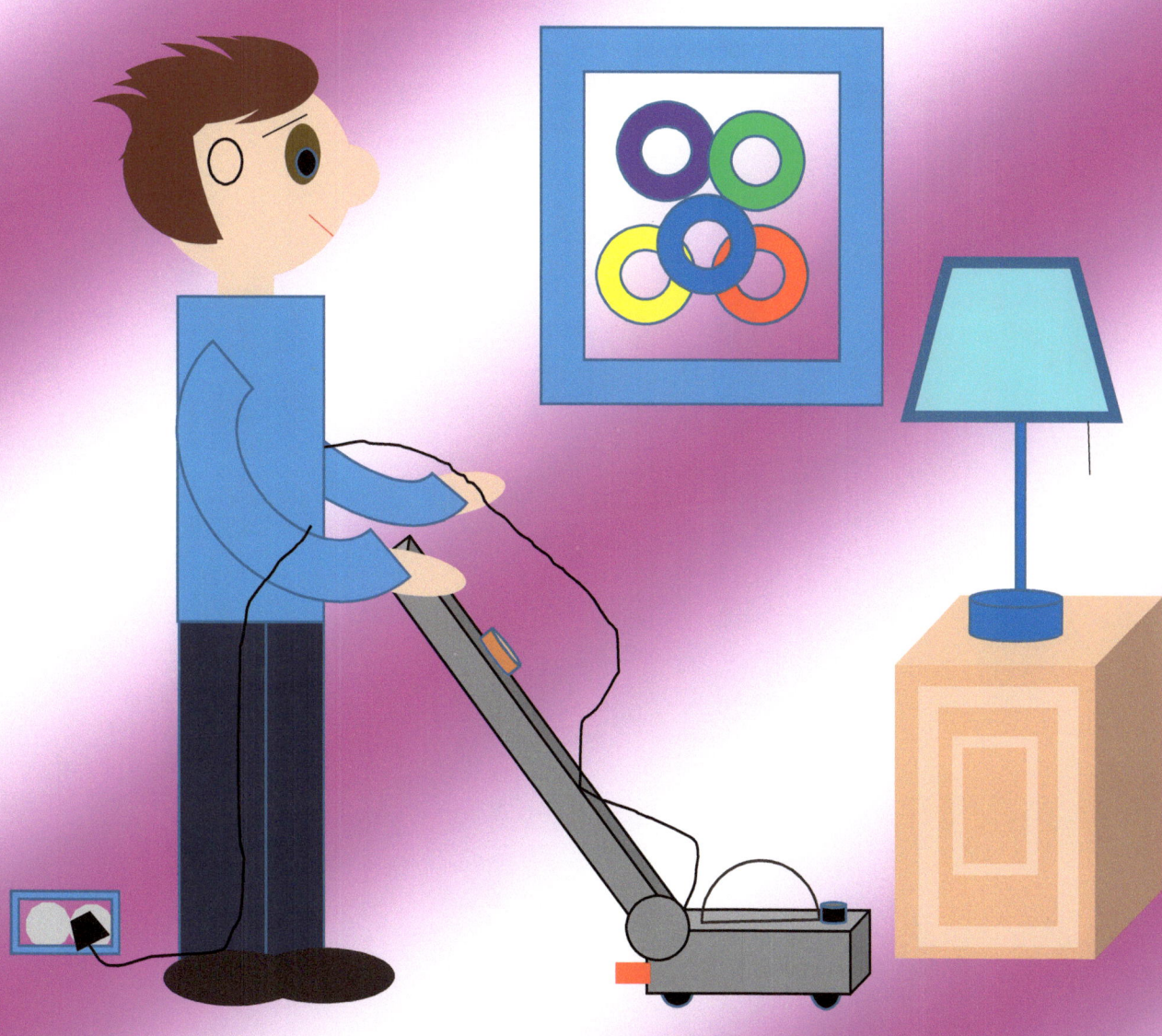

We want momma to eat healthy too!
Sometimes she doesn't feel like eating.
We make sure she drinks lots of
water.

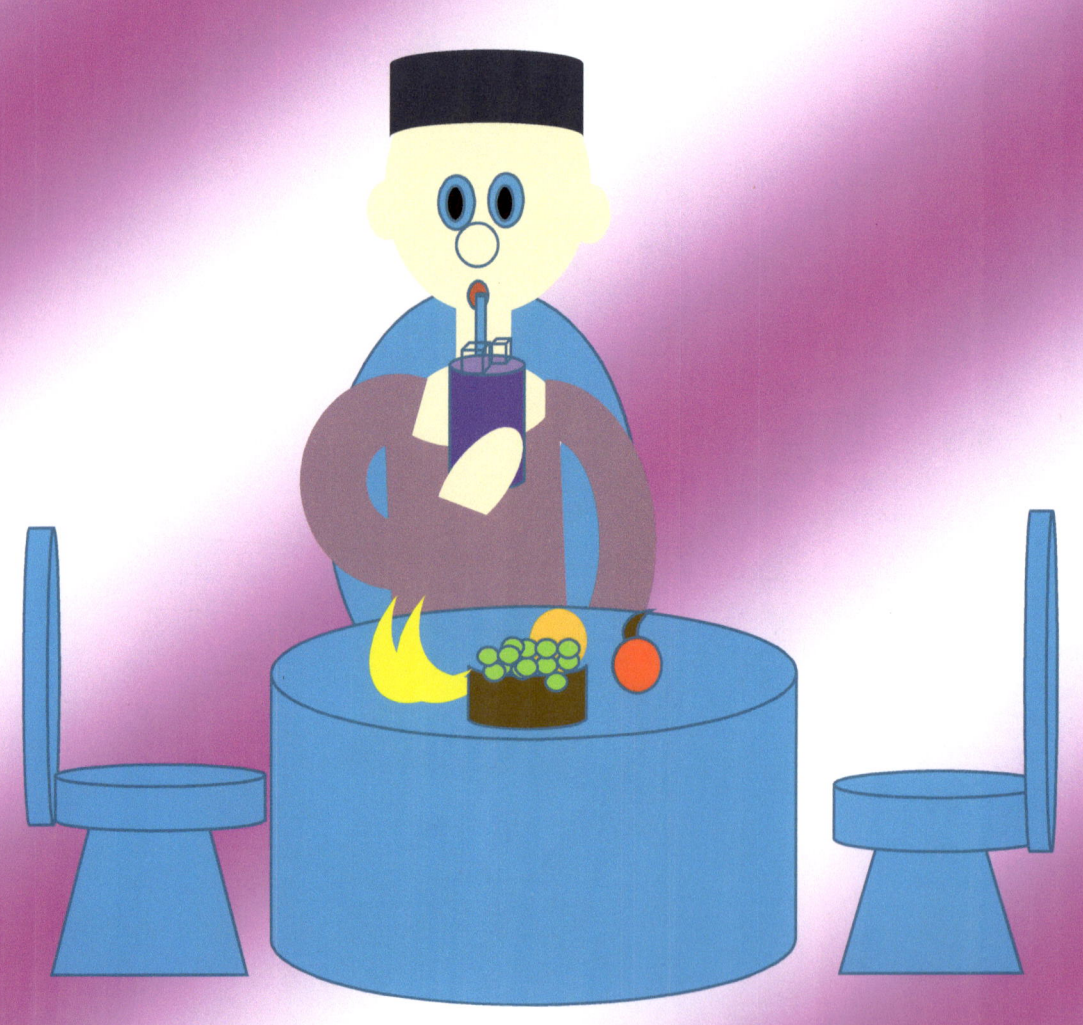

Momma falls asleep sometimes when we watch a movie together. We don't mind, she needs her rest.

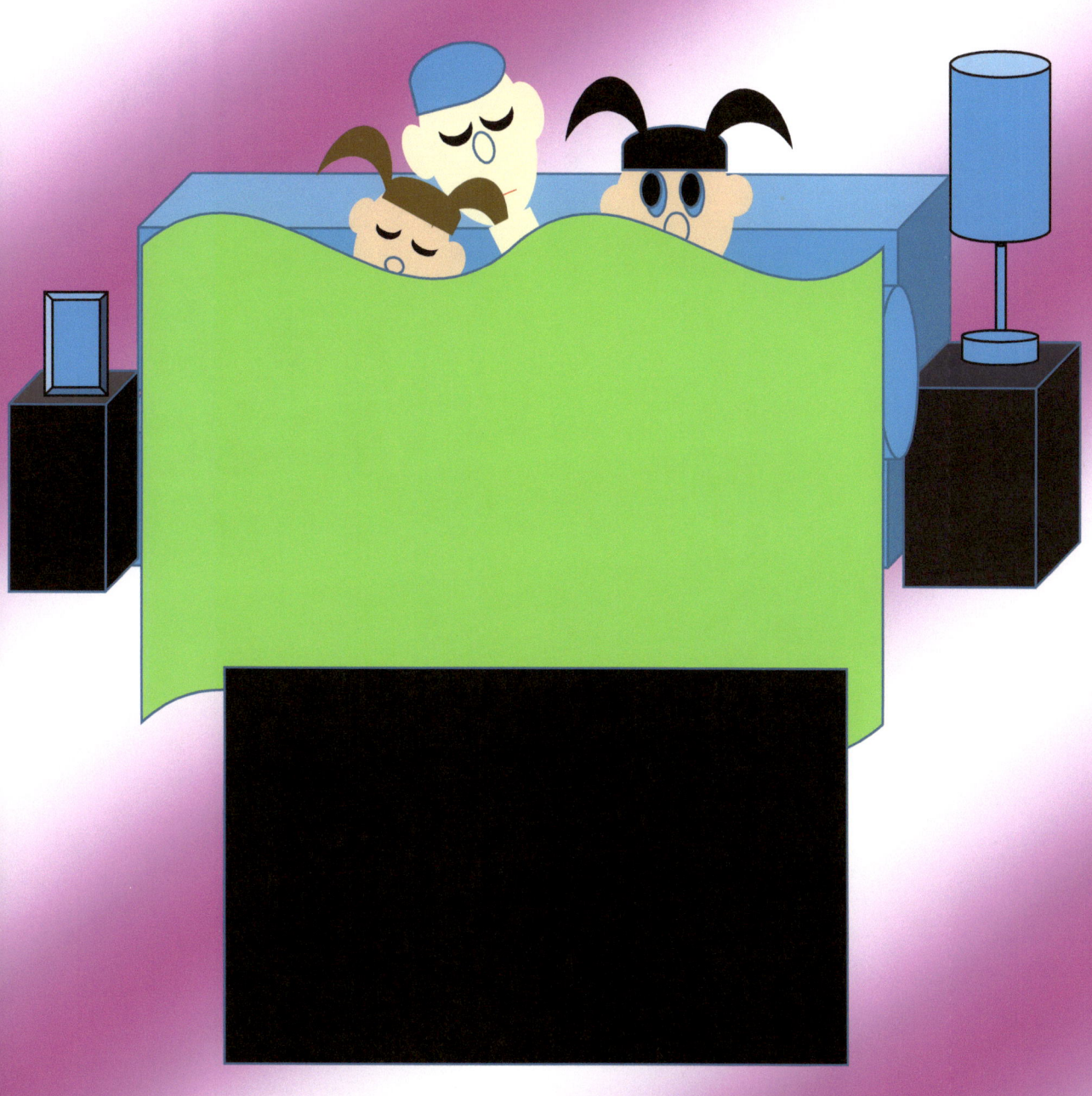

I'm not embarrassed. My momma has cancer. She still is my momma. She is sick and is doing what she can to get better. I love her, always.

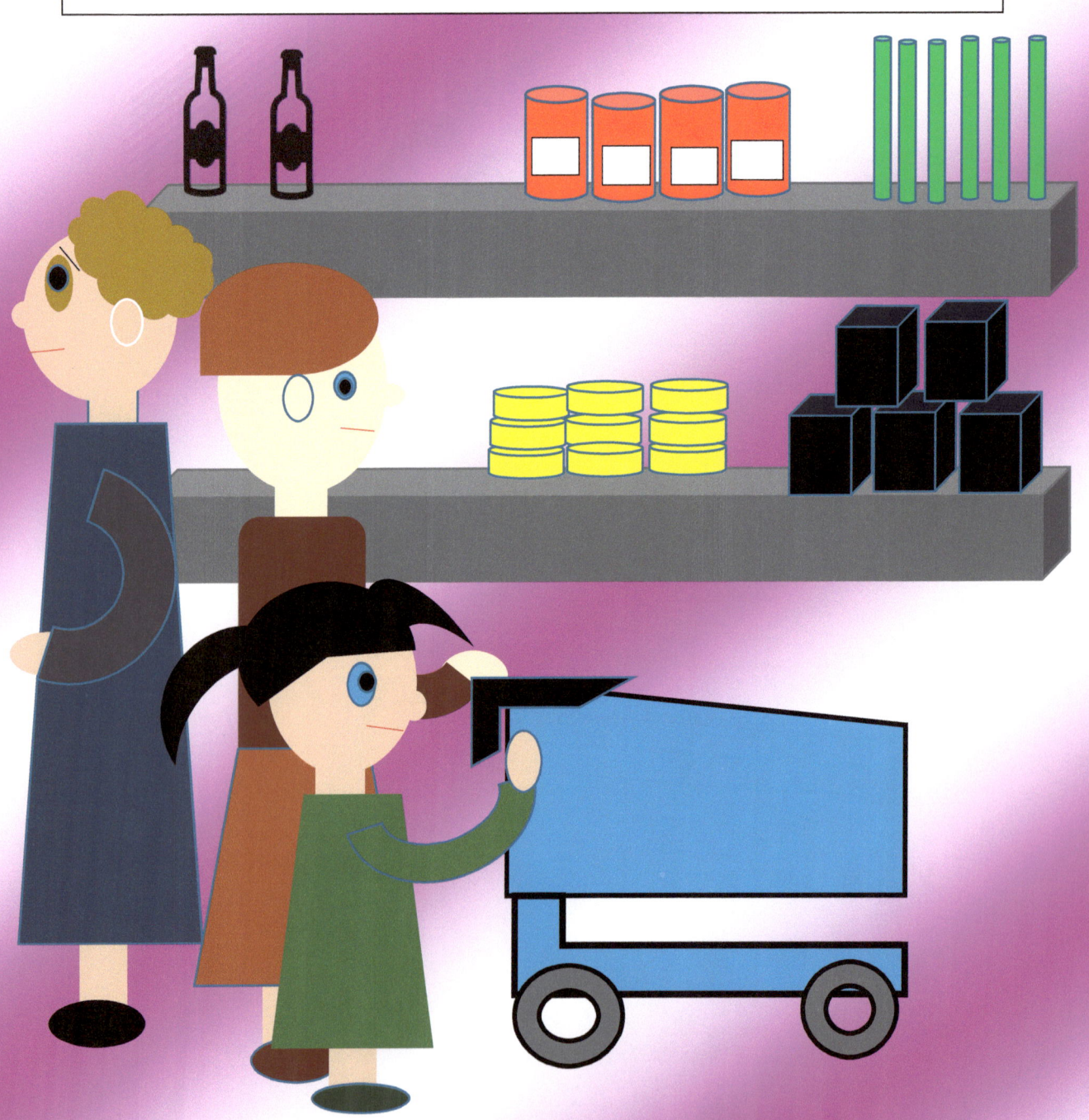

I told my friends about momma. Kaylie said "That's scary." Hallie said "She's going to die." Elle said nothing. She just stared at me. I felt bad.

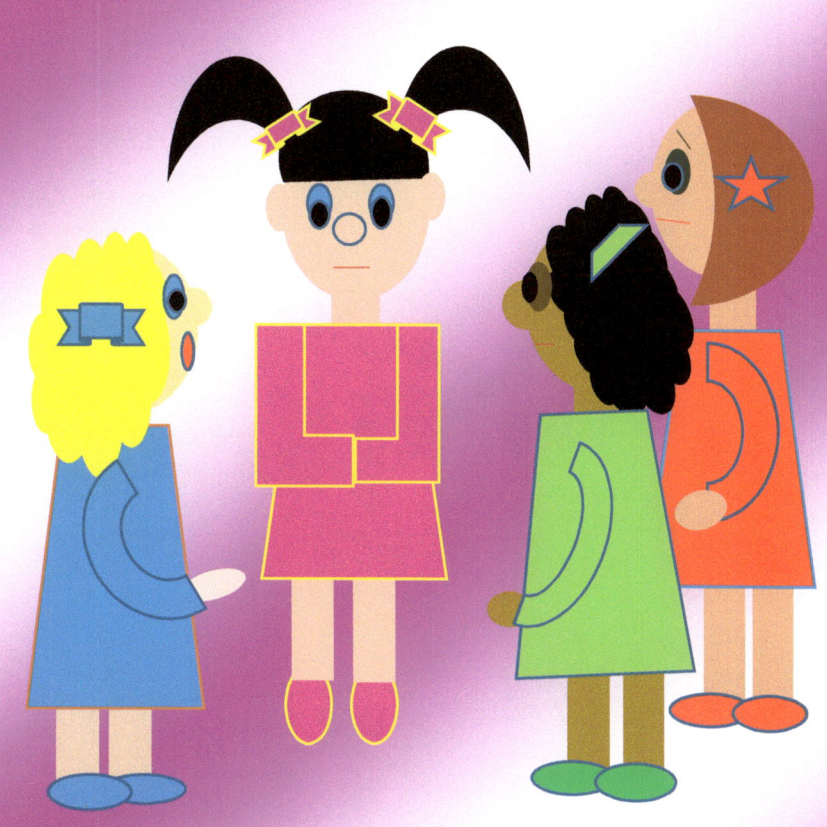

I cried at school. My teacher said she knew about momma. I told her what my friends said. She said "Sweetie, sometimes people just don't know what to say. They don't understand cancer. Don't be upset, they just don't understand."

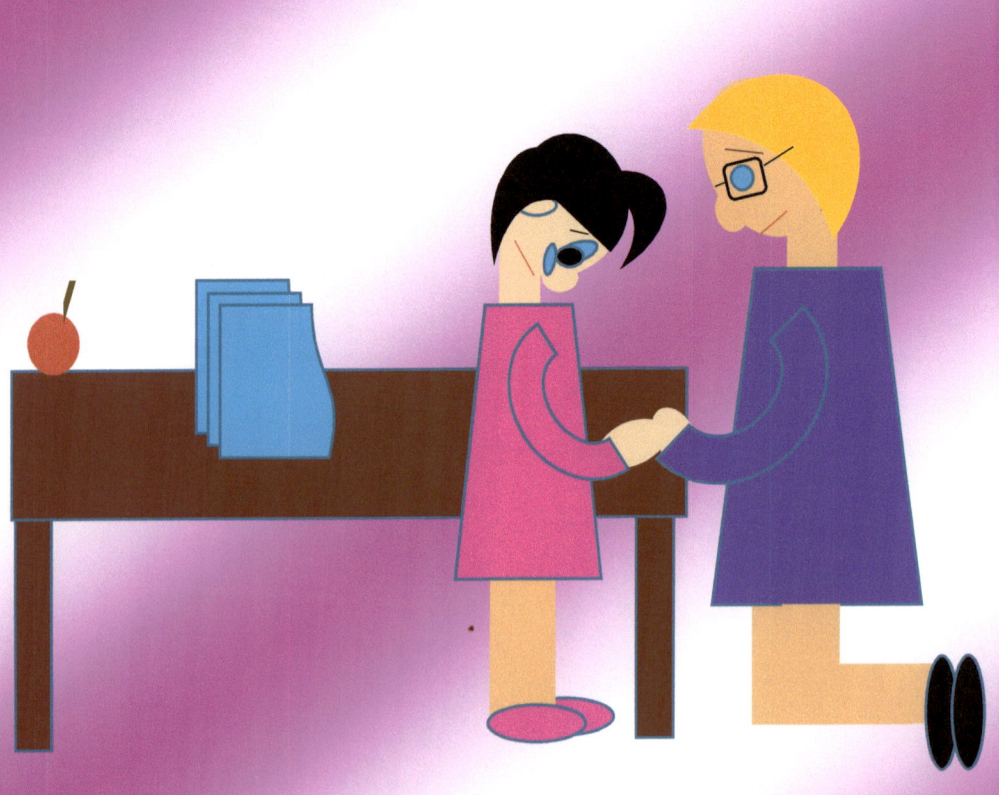

A lot of people come over and give us food. I like that. That is so nice. Others come over to help watch us. I guess they want to help us. People can be very nice.

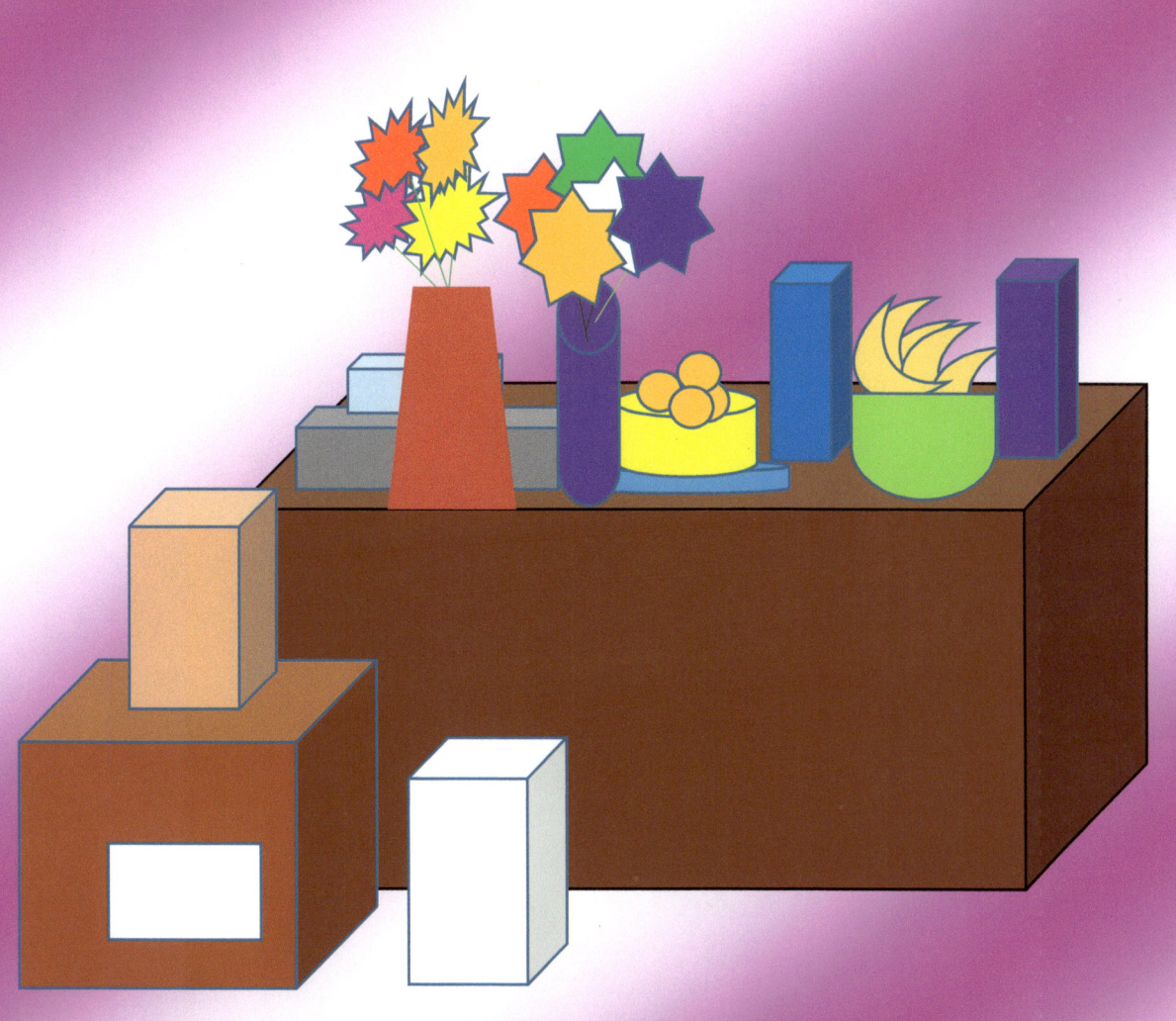

So, all I can tell you is cancer can be scary. It is what it is. You can help in many ways. Talk to your parents. When you know about it, it isn't as scary.

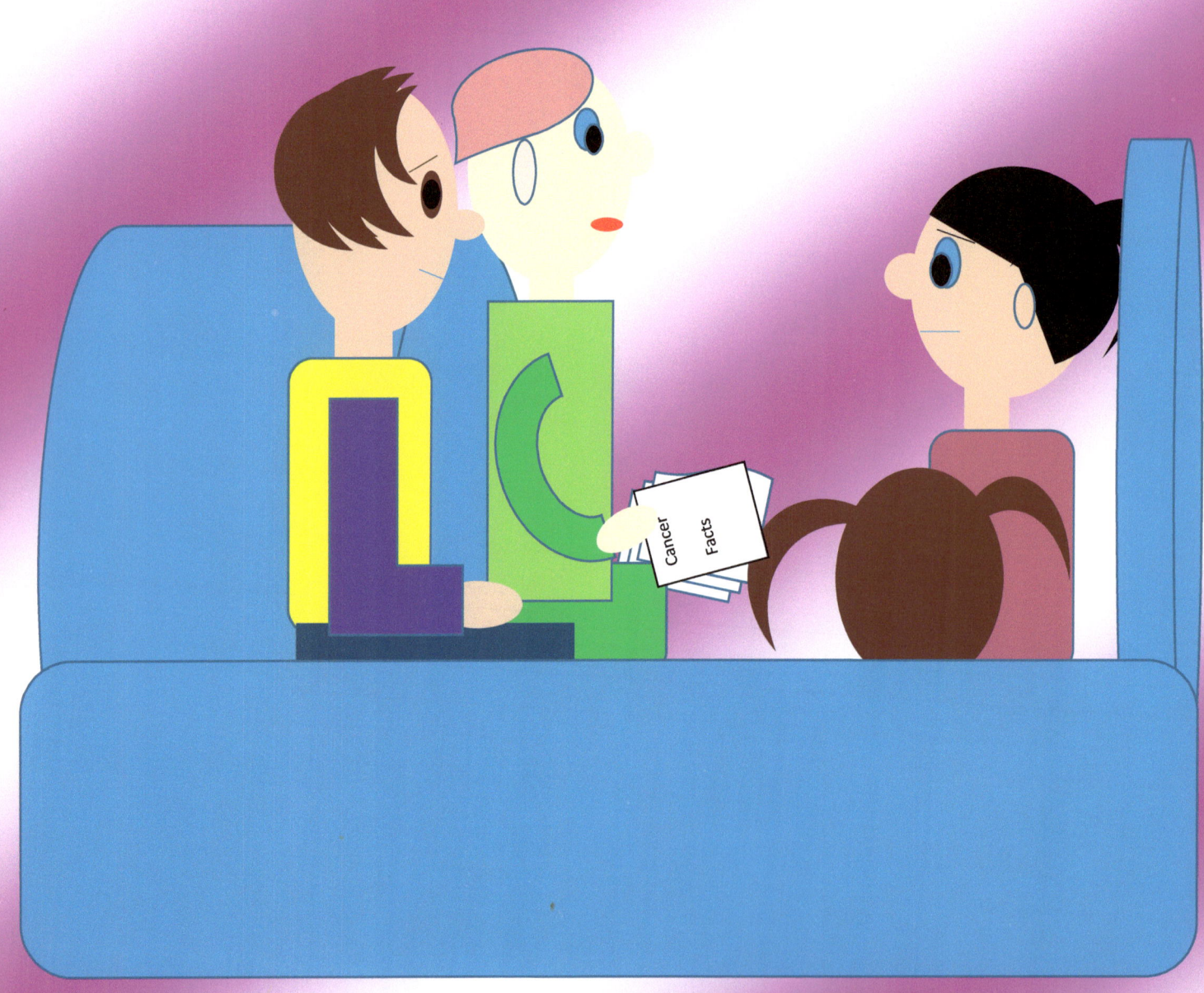

Momma said it was important for me to be strong, but it was okay to cry if I felt sad. Sometimes we laughed and cried together.

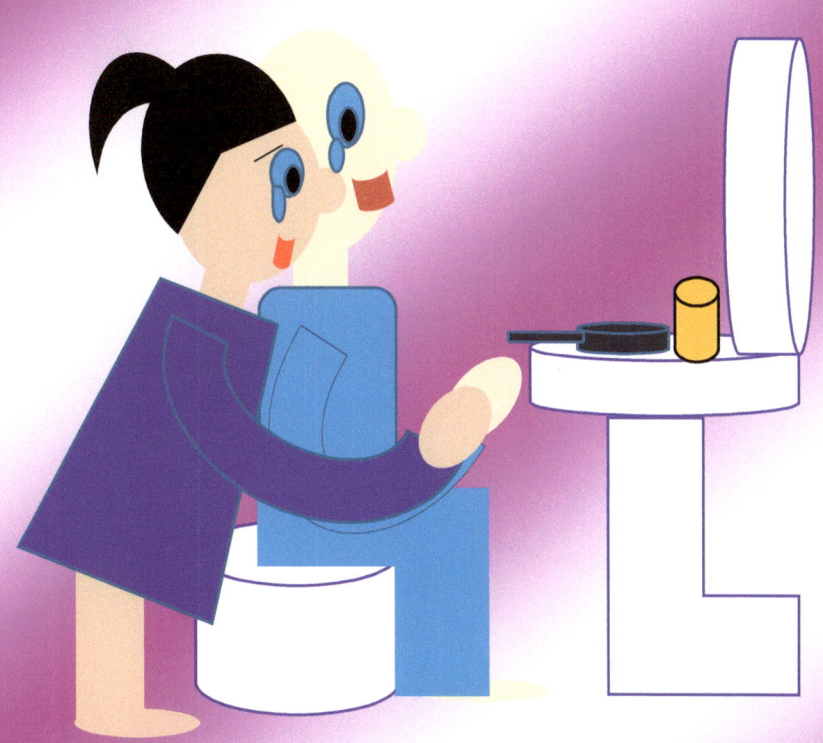

When my Aunt Cee had cancer, she died. Sometimes that does happen. Momma said we all are going to die someday. It's okay. What is important is how we live.

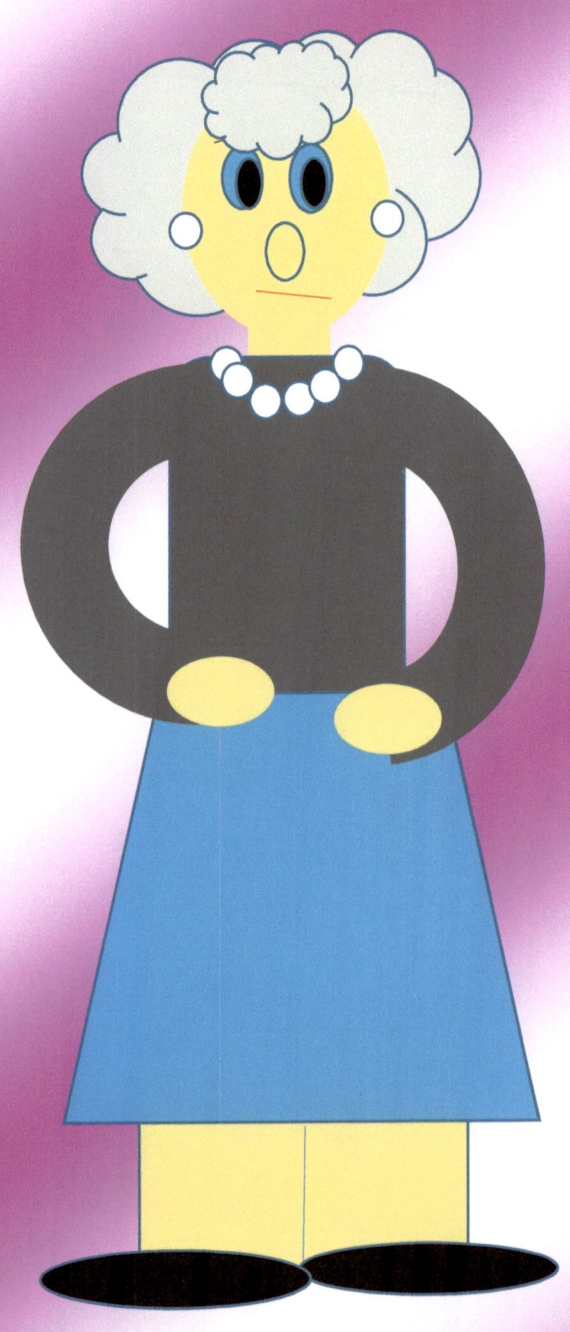

Momma said "Be happy in all that you do, be kind and loving."

It's not easy, I get mad at my sister when she breaks my toys. I still love her but I don't always like her.

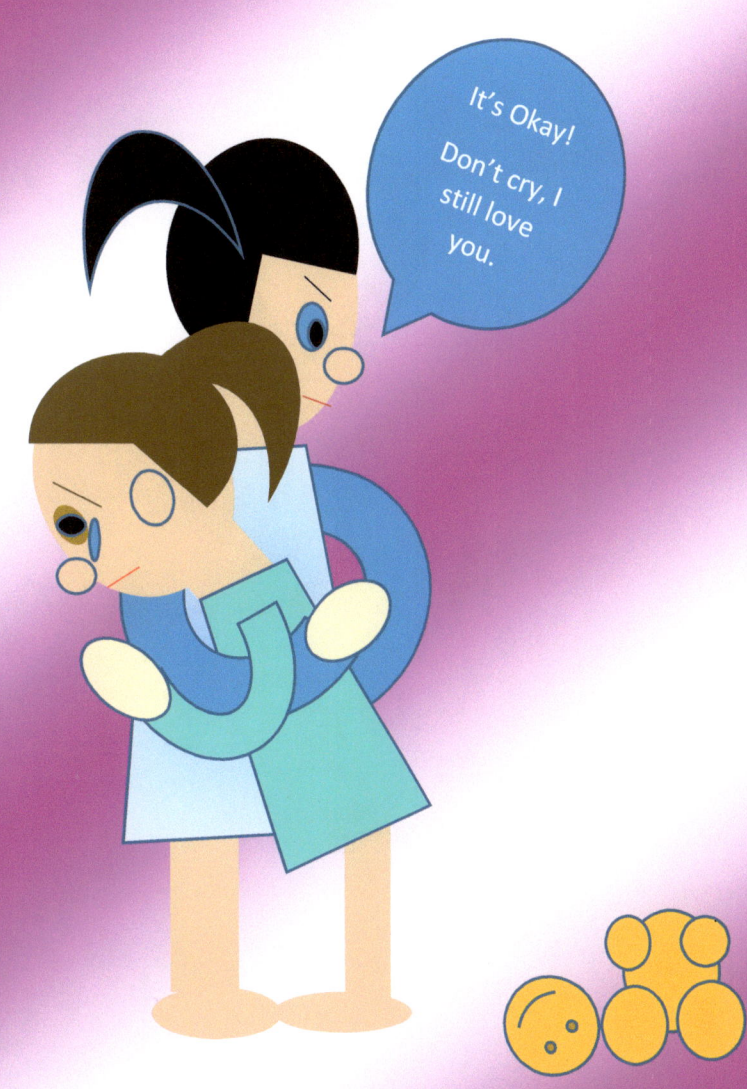

Momma said cancer had her, but we scared it away. It's important to not let it scare you. We are ok. We have each other.

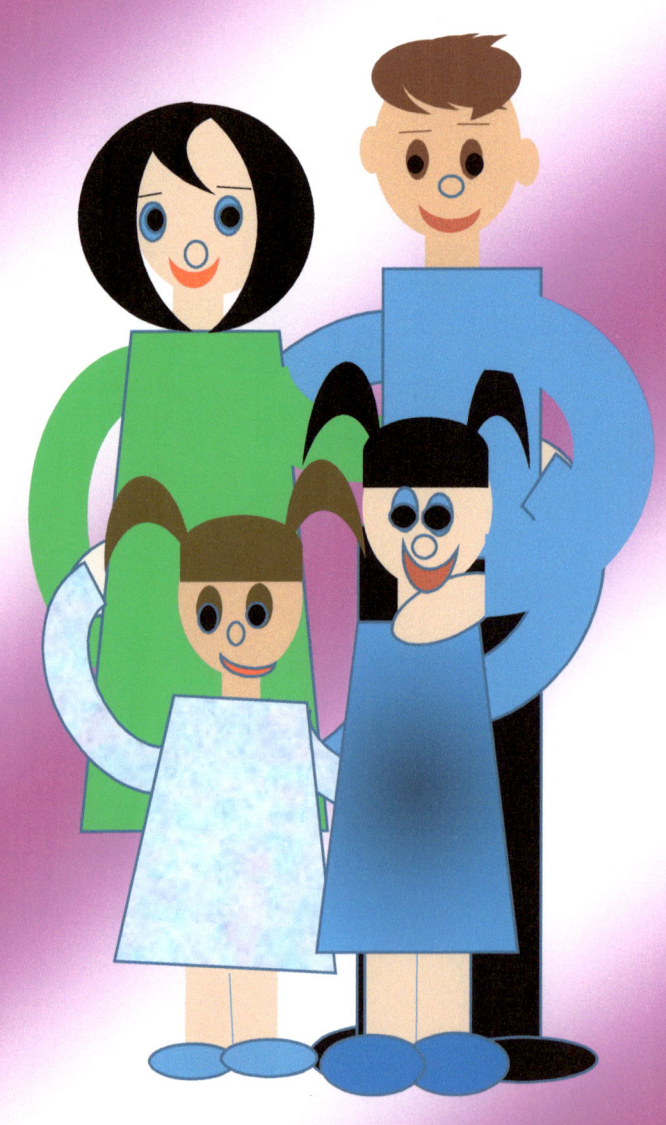

Other books by this Author:

Harry Is Okay

My Brother Riley

Just Different

Could You Repeat That, C.A.P.D

Anxiety

Autism? No, Really, What Is It?

Life Skills Social Stories I (home)

Life Skills Social Stories II (school)

The "B's" of Bullying

A Cat Named Dog

A Way Around Rude

Really?

I'm Confused America!

Christian Series

Where Is God?

I Can't Sleep At Night

On Papa's Lap

http://pacedpatience.wixsite.com/pacedpatience

Amazon.com or Createspace estore

found under Laura Vercillo or

Paced Patience.

https://www.teacherspayteachers.com/Store/Paced-Patience

www.ingramcontent.com/pod-product-compliance
Lightning Source LLC
Chambersburg PA
CBHW041310180526
45172CB00003B/1041